Table of Contents

INTRODUCTION

Congratulations on purchasing this book and thank you for doing so. This book is designed specifically for those who want to learn the basics of bariatric surgery and learn how to prepare simple and tasty recipes for each stage of recovery following bariatric surgery.

Bariatric surgery is very effective and brings results. However, to get the best results, it is important to fully understand the process and not lose the intricate and important details.

The purpose of this book is to explain how to make easy, healthy and delicious recipes for each stage of recovery before and after bariatric surgery using simple ingredients.

This book will not only teach you how to make your own recipes, it will also explain in detail how you can move towards better health.

I hope you will make the most of this book.

There are many books on this subject on the market, thank you again for choosing this one! Every effort has been made to ensure that it is full of as much useful information as possible; enjoy it!

CHAPTER 1 - BARIATRIC SURGERY

Obesity and Bariatric Surgery

Obesity is a chronic condition often difficult to treat with a simple diet combined with regular exercise. In these cases, bariatric surgery is a valid therapeutic option, especially for severely obese people suffering from serious health problems aggravated by excess weight.

Bariatric surgery includes a variety of procedures that promote weight loss by reducing food intake and/or absorption. Weight loss can be achieved by reducing the size of the stomach with a gastric band, by surgical resection (partial vertical gastrectomy or biliopancreatic diversion with duodenal switch) or by creating a small gastric pocket directly connected to a section of the small intestine (gastric bypass and variants). The best outcome is obtained when the patient undergoing surgery is strongly determined to follow strict dietary guidelines and to perform regular physical activity after surgery. In addition, the subject must also agree to long-term commitment to follow-up and post-operative medical treatment. These behaviours are essential to maintain the results obtained with bariatric surgery.

Who can resort to Bariatrics surgery?

At present, bariatric surgery is a suitable option for patients who:

- They have severe obesity.
- Have failed to achieve effective results with a controlled feeding programme (with or without pharmacological support).
- Have associated diseases such as hypertension, reduced glucose tolerance, diabetes mellitus, hyperlipidaemia and obstructive sleep apnea.

To define obesity levels, the body mass index (BMI) is used, an indicator of the shape weight status that relates to an individual's height and weight. An individual with BMI $\geq$ 30 is considered obese.

Bariatric surgery is only recommended for people with at least one of the following characteristics:

- BMI > 40 (class III/extremely severe obesity).
- BMI> 35 (class II/severe obesity), associated with at least one obesity-related pathological condition that can improve with weight loss.

However, recent research suggests that bariatric surgery may also be appropriate for people with a BMI of 35-40 without associated disease or with a BMI of 30-35 and significant comorbidities.

Anyone considering bariatric surgery to achieve significant weight loss should be aware of the risks and benefits of treatment.

The patient can be considered eligible for bariatric surgery if:

- Cannot achieve or maintain a beneficial level of weight loss (for at least six months) by adopting appropriate non-surgical solutions, such as diet, medications and exercise.
- He agrees to make a long-term commitment, after surgery, to a healthy diet and regular physical activity; he is therefore aware of the limits he will have to place on his future dietary choices and the need for regular follow-up.
- It has no medical or psychological obstacles to surgery or use of anaesthesia and does not abuse alcohol and/or drugs.
- He is motivated to improve his health and is aware of how life can change after surgery (for example, patients must adapt to side effects, such as the need to chew food well or the inability to eat large amounts of food).

There is no safe method, including surgery, to produce significant weight loss and maintain it over time. Some people who undergo bariatric surgery may experience a weight loss lower than expected; others may regain some of the weight lost over time. This recovery may vary according to the degree of obesity and the type of surgery. Some bad habits, such as lack of exercise or frequent consumption of high calorie snacks, can also affect the long-term outcome of treatment.

What is the intragastric balloon and in which cases is it offered to the patient?

It is a non-surgical technique, performed by endoscopy and without anaesthesia, performed in an outpatient clinic or, at most, with a couple of days of hospitalization. A balloon, the BIB, is placed inside the stomach. This, when dilated, gives the patient a sense of satiety even with modest amounts of food. It should be removed after six months and is usually used before surgery. If necessary, once the balloon has been removed, and after a necessary period, the procedure can be repeated.

The positioning of the intragastric balloon can be proposed before bariatric surgery in cases of major obesity, with BMI>50, to try to lose weight while waiting for the surgery. Most bariatric patients, however, go directly to surgery after a period of evaluation and follow-up to assess their motivation.

For patients who refuse bariatric surgery, or who are unsuitable for surgery, an intragastric balloon may be chosen.

Classification Bariatric Procedures

Bariatric procedures can be grouped into three main categories:

1.   Malabsorption surgery. Malabsorptive surgical procedures reduce the absorption of food. They result in an irreversible reduction in the size of the stomach and their effectiveness derives mainly from the creation of a physiological condition: the gastric cavity is connected to the terminal part of the small intestine, which limits the absorption of calories and nutrients.

- They belong to this type:
- Biliopancreatic diversion (wider form of gastric bypass, with the gastric pocket joined to the ileum. It produces the most extreme malabsorption).
- Fasting aileal bypass.

2.   Restrictive procedures. The gastric restrictive surgery limits the introduction of food through a prevalent mechanical action. They are based on the formation of a small gastric pocket in the upper part of the stomach,

which limits the gastric volume and leaves the food channel in continuity through a narrow, non-dilatable orifice. The restrictive procedures act to reduce the amount of food taken orally.

- They belong to this type:
- Adjustable gastric bandage.
- Vertical gastroplasty.
- Sleeve gastrectomy (partial vertical gastrectomy).
- Intragastric balloon (non-surgical transient treatment).

3.   Mixed surgery. Mixed bariatric procedures apply both techniques simultaneously, as in the case of gastric bypass or sleeve gastrectomy with duodenal switch.

The type of surgery that more than any other can help an obese person depends on several factors. Patients should discuss with the referring surgeon which option is best suited to their needs.

Bariatric surgery can be performed using standard "open" approaches, which include laparotomy with abdominal wall incision, or laparoscopy. With the second technique, doctors insert surgical instruments through small cuts made in the abdomen, guided by a small camera that transmits the images to a monitor. Currently, in most cases laparoscopic bariatric procedures are performed because they are minimally invasive, require smaller incisions, create less tissue damage and are associated with fewer post-operative problems. However, not all patients are suitable for laparoscopy. Patients who are extremely obese (e.g. >350kg), who have undergone previous stomach surgery or who have complex health problems (severe heart and lung disease) may require the open approach.

Surgery options

There are four types of operations most performed: adjustable gastric bandage (AGB), Roux-en-Y gastric bypass (RYGB), biliopancreatic diversion with duodenal switch (BPD-DS) and vertical sleeve gastrectomy (or sleeve gastrectomy, VSG).

Adjustable gastric band (AGB): gastro restrictive surgery that reduces food intake by placing an elastic silicone band around the upper portion of the stomach. Lap band LAGB gastric band This creates a small gastric pocket that communicates with the rest of the stomach through a narrow, non-expandable emptying orifice. The containment capacity of the gastric pocket can be adjusted according to the patient's needs without resorting to further surgery; the bandage houses a saline solution that can be increased or decreased, varying its constrictive effect, by means of a thin catheter connecting to a reservoir placed just under the skin.

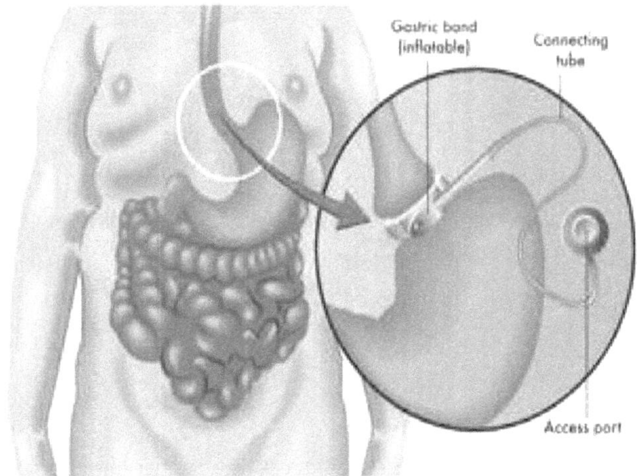

Weight loss is mainly due to the limited amount of food that can be ingested in a single meal (early satiety) and the increased time needed to digest the food introduced. It is often performed by laparoscopy (LAGB) and represents a reversible surgery: the gastric cavity is not sectioned, and the dressing can be removed. Weight loss: about 50% of the excess weight.

Roux-en-Y gastric bypass (RYGB): it is a mixed surgery, which limits both the intake and absorption of food. Roux-en-Y gastric bypass. The amount of food that can be ingested is limited by reducing (by surgical resection) the stomach to a small bag, similar in size to the pocket created with the gastric bandage. In addition, this small bag is connected, by means of a digestive loop, directly to the small intestine (at the level of the fast), excluding the digestive tract responsible for the absorption of nutrients (part of the stomach, duodenum and biliary tract). RYGB is considered an irreversible intervention, but in some cases the procedure can be partially reversed. Weight loss: about 60-70% of excess weight.

Roux-en-Y Gastric Bypass (RNY)

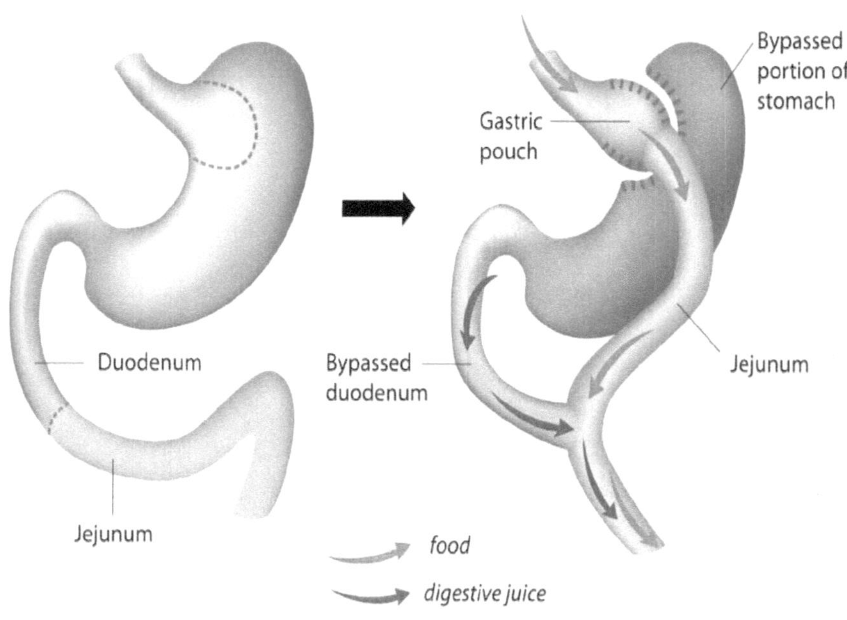

Biliopancreatic diversion with duodenal switch (BPD-DS): usually referred to as "duodenal switch" (duodenal inversion), it is a complex bariatric surgery with three peculiarities: Biliopancreatic diversion with duodenal switch1) it eliminates a large portion of the stomach (vertical resection), making patients prematurely satiated, who are "forced" to eat less; 2) it is a malabsorption surgery, where food is diverted and limited in its absorption: the surgeon creates a new food channel, creating an anastomosis between the residual gastric cavity and a small intestine tract (ileum); 3) the functionality of bile, pancreatic juice and enteric juices is modified, affecting the body's ability to digest the elements and absorb calories.

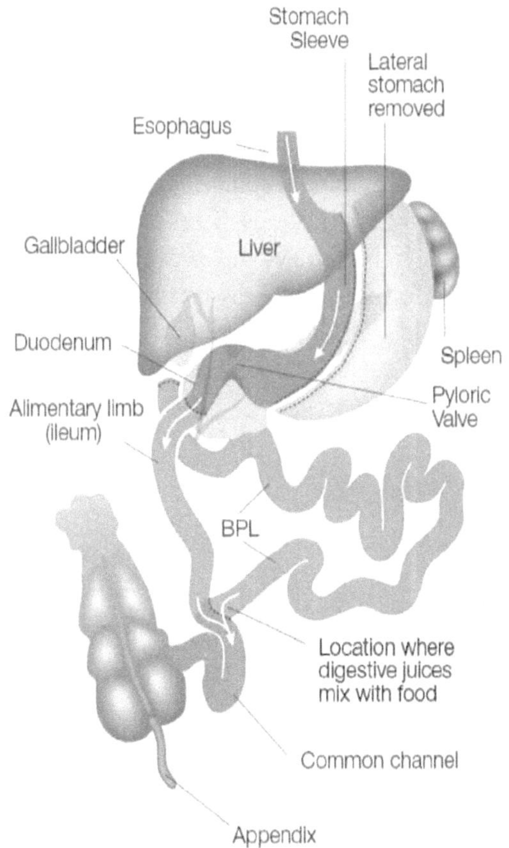

This operation leaves a small part of the available duodenum needed to absorb food, vitamins and minerals. However, when the patient ingests a meal, most of the intestine is bypassed (this is a more "drastic operation than the previous one"). The distance between the stomach and colon becomes much shorter after this operation, thus limiting the normal way in which food is absorbed. BPD-DS produces significant weight loss (about 65-75% of excess weight). However, a decrease in the amount of nutrients, vitamins and minerals absorbed leads to a high risk of long-term complications (anaemia, osteoporosis, etc.). For this reason, biliopancreatic diversion is generally only recommended when it is considered that rapid weight loss is essential to avoid a serious health condition, such as heart disease.

Partial vertical gastrectomy (VSG, vertical sleeve gastrectomy): belongs to gastro restrictive surgery because it limits food intake by reducing the size of the stomach.

Partial vertical gastrectomy This form of bariatric surgery is used for the treatment of severely obese people (BMI $\geq$ 60) for whom a bandage or gastric bypass is not recommended. In such circumstances, both procedures would carry a very high risk of causing complications. The aim of the procedure is to induce an early sense of satiety. To achieve this, a partial vertical resection of 80-90% of the stomach is performed during the procedure. The weight loss should be about 60%. Once this result has been achieved, it should be possible to perform a gastric bandage or bypass safely.

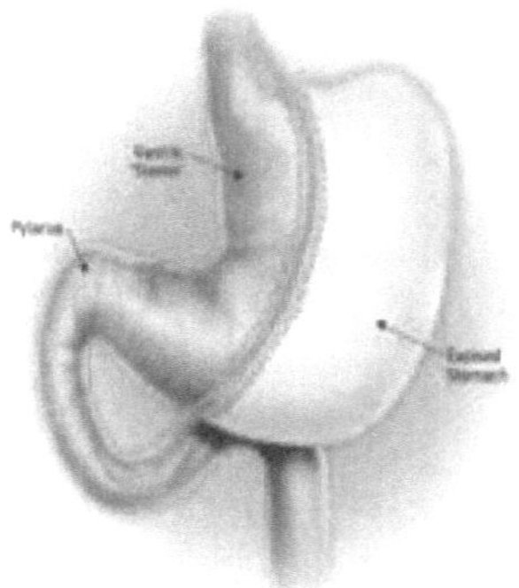

The patient and the competent surgeon have to confront each other in order to choose the best surgical option, evaluating the long-term effects and possible complications that may arise during and after the operation (such as problems related to malabsorption, vomiting and oesophageal reflux, the inability to eat abundant meals, the need to limit especially certain foods, etc.). Other factors to consider are the patient's BMI, his eating habits, the repercussions of obesity on his health and any previous stomach surgery.

The aim of bariatric surgery is to reduce the risk of illness or death associated with obesity. In general, malabsorption procedures lead to greater weight loss than restrictive procedures but have a higher risk profile.

After Surgery

How long is the hospital stay after surgery?

Generally, after a gastric bandage two to three days are enough. This is different from the case of the gastrectomy sleeve, which requires one day of pre-recovery and four or five days of hospitalization.

How do you evaluate the success of the operation, in the so-called "follow-up" phase?

First, the follow-up after bariatric surgery consists of a series of dietary, dietary, psychological and surgical evaluations over a year. Contact with the dietician and the psychologist must be constant, while the surgeon's check-ups take place after one, three, six months and then after a year. The check-ups continue even beyond that, to assess any nutritional deficiencies resulting, for example, in iron or vitamin levels.

Recovery after bariatric surgery

Immediately after bariatric surgery, the patient is restricted to a liquid diet, which includes foods such as broth or diluted fruit juices. This line is adopted until the complete recovery of the gastrointestinal tract from the operation. In the subsequent stages, the patient is "forced" to take only modest amounts of food, since if he exceeds the stomach's capacity to contain it, he may experience nausea, headache, vomiting, diarrhoea, dysphagia, etc. The dietary restrictions partly depend on the type of surgery. Many patients, for example, will need to take one multivitamin a day for life to compensate for the reduced absorption of essential nutrients.

Side Effects

A variety of complications can be associated with bariatric surgery procedures. The risks depend on the type of surgery and any other health problems present before the operation. In postoperative surgery, some short-term complications (within 1-6 weeks after surgery) may include bleeding, surgical wound infection, bowel obstruction, nausea and vomiting (due to excess food or stenosis at the surgical site). Other problems that may occur are related to nutrient deficiencies, typical of people undergoing poorly absorbing bariatric procedures that do not take vitamins and minerals; in extreme cases, if patients do not cope with the problem, diseases such as pellagra (caused by vitamin B3 deficiency, niacin), pernicious anaemia (vitamin B12 deficiency) and beri (caused by vitamin B1 thiamine deficiency) may occur. After bariatric surgery, other important medical complications may include venous thromboembolism (deep vein thrombosis in the legs and pulmonary embolism), heart attack, pneumonia, urinary tract infections, gastrointestinal ulcers, gastric and/or intestinal fistula, stenosis and hernias (laparocele and internal hernia).

CHAPTER 2 – GASTRIC SLEEVE DIET

Diet Before Surgery

Food restrictions begin at least two weeks before the day of the operation to help the body cope with it. The diet prepares the digestive tract and liver for the operation and helps the body prepare for lifestyle changes that affect the diet.

Foods to limit or avoid:

- Fried foods
- Fatty foods
- Desserts and sweets
- Sugar
- alcohol
- carbonated beverages
- made with whole milk.

Food to eat:

- yogurt
- oatmeal
- ricotta
- lean meat
- sugar-free jelly
- wholemeal foods
- oatmeal
- scrambled eggs only albumen
- protein shakes

We must say goodbye to binge drinking and welcome three small, well-balanced meals. Two of these meals will be protein shakes and for dinner you can eat lean meat, salad, etc. Protein is essential in the preoperative diet because it allows the body to get rid of fat.

Meals must be eaten at the right time and, in order to prevent blockage, the food consumed must be chewed carefully until it has a pasty consistency. In addition to drinking plenty of water, the patient is advised to avoid coffee and carbonated beverages. Drugs, such as non-steroidal anti-inflammatory drugs and medicinal herbs, should be avoided one week before surgery. In addition, 8 hours before surgery, the patient should not consume anything.

After surgery diet

Immediately after surgery the patient may feel nauseous but may consume fluids to avoid dehydration. Among them:

- water
- green tea
- broth
- sugar-free jelly
- sugar-free popsicles
- ice cubes

The liquids must be sipped very slowly and as soon as he feels full, the patient must stop drinking. He should never use a straw, because if he drinks too much his stomach may expand.

After two weeks: Semi-liquid diet

The patient is not yet allowed to consume soft or solid foods, as solid foods may break the staples in the stomach and thus increase the risk of spillage.

The recommended liquids are:

- broth
- green tea
- diluted juices
- skimmed milk
- water
- soya milk

- low-fat soups
- yoghurt light
- protein drinks
- sugar-free jelly

After 3/8 weeks

Due to the danger of paperclips breaking, the patient is asked to consume only baby food and milkshake. In addition, pieces of food may get stuck in the opening of the stomach and cause excruciating pain and vomiting.

Only milkshake or mashed foods are allowed at this stage:

- poultry and meat milkshakes
- milkshakes
- fish or scallops
- boiled vegetable cream

After 9/12 weeks

The patient is now ready for soft food. Almost all foods on the list of soft foods are allowed, provided they are low in sugar and fat, such as:

- oatmeal
- sugarless pudding
- scrambled eggs
- low-fat ricotta
- cooked vegetables and milkshakes
- baked fish without bones

Protein foods are recommended. In addition, it should take 4-5 hours from one meal to the next. Each meal should last at least thirty minutes and should include only a few snacks.

After 4 months: Soft Diet

The patient's diet is becoming more regular.

Lean meat, poached eggs, fruit, vegetables, cereals.

Rice, pasta and bread may still not be tolerated due to their high starch content, so they should be avoided. It should be remembered that the amounts a patient can consume are very small and will feel full after eating only a few bites. This promotes weight loss. It is important not to consume food and liquids at the same time.

After 2 years

After the first two years of surgery, the diet is restricted to 600-800 calories per day. The weight is lost more during the first year. After the gastrectomy, the recommended diet will vary from person to person; foods will be added or removed from the diet, depending on the level of tolerance. Before and after the surgery, the patient should maintain regular physical activity to maximize weight loss. Once the appropriate weight is reached, calorie intake increases to 1000 - 1200 calories per day.

People who have undergone a gastrectomy will have to eat small amounts throughout their lives and will have to avoid high-calorie foods, carbonated drinks, etc. The diet will be specified in the hospital and all instructions given by the professional doctor must be strictly followed.

Recommended Foods

Milk: Preferably use low-fat milk and yoghurt.

Bread: Use wholemeal or plain bread. Prefer wholemeal foods. Exclude bread with oil, milk or seasoned bread in general.

Pasta: Use pasta, rice, semolina, barley and corn flour. Long pasta and wholemeal rice recommended. Limit once a week the use of egg or stuffed pasta (ravioli, tortellini) and gnocchi. It can cook in degreased meat or vegetable broth. Use simple sauces: tomato, mushrooms, vegetables, avoiding elaborate sauces with high caloric density (cream, bacon, sausage, etc..).

Meat: Use beef, horse, rabbit, turkey, chicken, veal, pork, lamb in the leanest parts and deprived of visible fat. The skin of the poultry must be removed before cooking. Cooking must be carried out without fat, which may be added raw at the end of cooking. Breading and fried must be excluded.

Fish: Use fresh or frozen lean fish (grouper, snapper, hake, cod, trout, perch, swordfish, sardines, turbot, gilthead bream, trout, mullet) Limit semi-fat fish (carp). Avoid first time fatty fish (eel, eel, eel, mackerel, salmon). Cook as for meat.

Cheese: Use two, three times a week at most. Prefer fresh cheese (crescenza, scamorza, fior di latte, provola, taleggio magro, quartirolo, ricotta, mozzarella).

Avoid the more mature and fatty cheeses (fontina, grana, asiago, belpaese, caciocavallo, caciotta toscana, caciotta di pecora, gorgonzola, emmenthal, fresh pecorino, sweet provolone, pastorella).

Cold cuts: Use a couple of times a week raw ham, naturally cooked, bresaola, lean speck carefully deprived of visible fat.

Eggs: Use two to four eggs per week (maximum). Cooking without fat. The egg is more digestible if after cooking the egg white is thick and the yolk soft (soft boiled, poached, steamed).

Vegetables: Use all types of vegetables: raw, cooked, varied as much as possible, with the exception of potatoes that will be eaten instead of pasta and bread and legumes that can be used as a source of protein for dishes with cereals (pasta and beans, barley and lentils, etc..).

Fruit: Use all fresh seasonal fruit, raw at least once a day, cooked, smoothed or pressed, varied as much as possible. Limit very sugary fruit (persimmons, bananas, figs, grapes). Avoid dried fruit (nuts, hazelnuts, peanuts, almonds, plums), fruit in syrup and chestnuts.

Seasonings: Use preferably extra virgin olive oil, or sunflower oil, soya beans or rice always raw. Limit the use of butter, always raw. Exclude margarine, lard and animal fats in general.

Gr. 10 of oil = 1 soup spoon.

Gr. 5 of oil = 1 tablespoon of tea.

Gr. 10 of oil = gr. 10 of butter.

Drinks: Allowed natural mineral water, tea and coffee but in moderate quantities. Exclude alcoholic drinks, sugars, carbonated beverages of all kinds (soft drinks, fruit juices, liqueurs, bitters, grappa, etc. ...).

Sweets: Exclude sweets of any kind (sugar, honey, jam, candy, chocolate, biscuits, ice cream, cakes, puddings and creams).

Miscellaneous: Exclude very fatty substances (mayonnaise, cocoa, cream, tuna sauce, olives, food in oil, preserved foods in general except frozen). Useful the use of aromatic herbs (parsley, sage, laurel, rosemary, etc..). Moderate use of spices (pepper, nutmeg, cinnamon, saffron, etc..).

Frequency, volume and duration of meals

The frequency of meals is very important. You should follow a daily distribution of meals divided into three main meals: breakfast, lunch and dinner and at least two to three daily snacks as needed.

The volume of meals should be limited: you should start - to re-hydrate - with about 150 ml at a time, corresponding to a glass of water; means can be used to adjust easily, such as a straw or a teaspoon. In addition to the volume of meals, it is important to recognize the volume of liquids and it is of fundamental importance not to drink while eating, regardless of the type of surgery you have undergone. In this way you do not overload your stomach and therefore avoid what are the possible consequences: vomiting and nausea. Liquids are taken half an hour before meals and after meals.

Another important factor is the duration of meals. People need to take the correct time to eat; this aspect is fundamental because it often happens that before the operation they eat in a hurry, a habit that is harmful to digestion. In the preoperative phase the patient is educated to eat slowly and chew carefully to avoid consequences that could be discomfort, vomiting and even intense nausea.

Another recommendation is to stop eating when they feel full, so as not to cause other problems and not to induce harmful dilation. The bites should be small, and the food cut into small pieces and the meal should last at least 20-30 minutes.

Food quality

People who have undergone bariatric surgery, for example gastric bypass surgery, know that after the operation there can be taste alterations that last over time. Also, in this case, it will be the individual who will have to orient themselves towards the foods considered most suitable for the palate. In general, however, all those foods that are rich in carbohydrates and fats should be eliminated.

White meat should be preferred over red meat because it is less fibrous and more digestible.

Vegetables should be cut thinly, favouring cooked ones rather than raw ones, at least initially.

Cooking must be simple, not too elaborate dishes.

What are the behaviours to avoid?

Here are some behaviours to avoid that every time we recommend to our patients to minimize any gastrointestinal discomfort.

- ➤ Lie down immediately after meals
- ➤ Eat fast
- ➤ Chew quickly and roughly food
- ➤ Drinking during meals
- ➤ Drinking carbonated drinks
- ➤ Drink less than a litre of natural water a day. In this regard, it is important to always remember that to maintain the right rehydration,

it is best not to exceed 100-150 ml at a time (1 glass of water).

Evaluation of micronutrient intake in the operated patient

The drastic reduction of ingested food leads the body to a deprivation of calories, macronutrients and micronutrients. In particular:

-Vitamin B12 because it is absorbed in the intestine thanks to a molecule, the intrinsic factor, which is produced in the stomach; a large component of the gastric wall is removed in the sleeve and especially if associated with a low intake of meat and / or dairy products, these conditions can lead to B12 deficiency (Although theoretically you can have a deficit, there are no long-term data). B12 deposits are large and deficits are usually described one year after surgery. In addition to B12, iron, calcium, potassium, vitamin B9 (folates), vitamin B1 (thiamine), vitamin B6, zinc, selenium and fat-soluble vitamins (A, D, E, K) should also be monitored. Being a topic of great importance, the prevention of nutritional deficits in post-operative will be dealt with in a separate article.

Nutritional Supplementation

This is another important aspect in the post-operative phase of bariatric surgery patients. This is because people suffering from pathological obesity may present nutritional deficiencies even before the operation because they have followed - perhaps for long periods - incorrect dietary choices and the micronutrients could be dispersed in the fatty tissue substances. In addition, bariatric surgery leads to a reduced intake of vitamins and trace elements, as for example in the case of gastric banding, where this phenomenon is due to the reduction in income; also in the case of the sleeve, where in addition to this phenomenon there is also the increased speed of bolus transit with a reduction in gastric acidity and the reduction of gastric cavity cells that produce the so-called "extrinsic factor" essential for the absorption of vitamin B12. With regard to gastric bypass, the clinical picture also weighs on the fact that in addition to being a restrictive intervention it is also a malabsorption surgery and therefore it is essential to take the supplements that are prescribed in the immediate post-operative.

As far as iron supplements are concerned, it is good to take them on an empty stomach, to favour their assimilation.

FAQ

How much weight did I lose after the surgery?

As with any treatment, surgical or not, everything will depend on the person. It is not a linear weight loss, but the excess weight will be gradually lost during the first year, although the percentage changes from person to person. The most common thing is to lose between 5 and 6 kg the first month. There are patients who continue with these numbers for a few months and others who lose up to 40% of the extra pounds since the third or fourth month. From 12 or 18 months onwards, the loss slows down, although patients have usually already managed to lose between 65 and 85% of the excess weight.

As we have seen, after bariatric surgery with bypass, weight loss is practically assured even if there is always a minimum failure rate. The cause may not be related to the surgery itself but to the food the patient continues to consume. In order for the results to be as expected and the excess pounds to be lost, it will be necessary to follow a diet established by the surgeon, but after a few months, it will be enough to change some eating habits to continue losing weight. If this effect is not produced, if you do not follow the diet recommended by the doctor and do not aim for a healthy and balanced diet, the operation will not be of much use, and you will not reach the established goal.

What is stapling of the stomach?

It is an endoscopic technique that uses the natural way, from the mouth through the oesophagus, and uses a new tool that allows you to "stitch", to suture the stomach from the inside.

What is the best diet after surgery?

Any surgery is a stressful event for the body. It is therefore necessary to have a rest period before returning to normal daily activities.

Here are 10 tips:

1. **Rest**: In the 48 hours following blepharoplasty surgery it is good to rest with your head slightly raised. Do things calmly, take advantage of these days to relax and recover physically.

2. **Drink plenty of water**: to recover any lost liquids and keep your body hydrated.

3. **Taste and variety in dishes**: enrich your dishes with colour and taste. Often after surgery, your appetite is reduced. Cooking tempting dishes helps to restore hunger and not feel sick, as well as nourish the body, which now more than ever needs energy to recover. A small suggestion: add some spices, such as turmeric, ginger, sage, rosemary or oregano. You will immediately give flavour and colour to your dish, as well as enrich it with other beneficial properties.

4. **Choose foods that are easy to digest**: avoid foods that are too high in calories, fat, sugar and salt and prefer vitamins, minerals, antioxidants and fibre. Avoid alcohol, carbonated drinks and fried foods.

5. **Antioxidants**: Many foods naturally possess antioxidant substances that can fight oxidative stress and inflammation, which often increase after surgery. A good way to distinguish them is to classify fruit and vegetables by colour: antioxidants are often also directly responsible for the colouring of vegetables.

So, let's find out:

- ✓ Orange-red foods, whose antioxidants are important for eyesight and skin: pumpkin, carrots, tomatoes, peppers, citrus fruits, pomegranate, peaches, melon, apricots ...
- ✓ Blue-violet foods, important for the urinary tract, vision and good circulation. Red grapes, blueberries and berries, radishes, radicchio, wild plum, aubergines...
- ✓ Green food, source of magnesium and folic acid, with positive effect on bones and teeth. Asparagus, broccoli, cauliflower, spinach, kiwi...

6. **Seasonality**: always prefer seasonal fruit and vegetables, it is certainly tastier and richer in nutrients.

7. **Cooking method**: to keep the antioxidant substances intact, less aggressive cooking methods such as steam cooking should be preferred. Avoid excessive exposure of food to air and light, vitamin C, for example, is quickly destroyed by exposure to the sun or cooking. Avoid burning food.

8. **Wholegrain cereals and legumes**: when eaten together they are an excellent complete dish. Whole grains are rich in fibre, which is essential for regulating digestion. Bran and germ, in fact, contain important nutrients, which are lost with refining. The skin of legumes is rich in polyphenols and saponins, precious allies against free radicals.

9. **Better fish than meat**: especially blue fish, rich in two essential omega-3 fatty acids: EPA and DHA. Avoid red meat especially if treated or full of hormones and preservatives.

10. **Raw vegetable oils**: extra virgin olive oil is preferable to animal fats.

What should I take to the hospital?

Here is what you should put in your bag, the day you go to hospital for hospitalisation:

- everything necessary for personal hygiene (toothbrush, toothpaste, soap, towels, etc.).
- underwear.
- pajamas/nightgown.
- tracksuit.
- closed non-slip slippers.
- handkerchiefs.
- coins for snack and beverage dispensers.
- books or magazines;
- a CD or Mp3 player or portable radio with headphones.

It is strongly discouraged to carry valuables or large sums of money.

Does the part of the stomach remove grow back after the operation?

No as mention in the surgery it is a permanent surgery. There is no chance to grow back removed the part and the surgery is not reversible at any condition.

Which person is qualified for surgery?

Bariatric surgery is chosen in all those cases where the condition of obesity constitutes a real risk for the health of the person. Nevertheless, the surgical option is not for everyone: specific requirements must be met.

The first selection is clinical and requires the following requirements to be met:

- In addition to the "normal" effects of obesity, there must be related complications such as hypertension, sleep disorders or forms of diabetes.
- body mass index equal to or greater than 30 (remember that BMI = weight (in kg) / height square (in metres).
- Ineffectiveness of traditional methods (diet followed by a specialist, physical activity).

Once the requirements have been verified, it is up to the medical team, which may include a surgeon, a psychologist, a nutritionist and other figures. The team aims to assess the pros and cons of the operation in relation to the specific characteristics of the person and if the potential benefits outweigh the potential risks, the green light is given.

The following are the elements that may influence the medical team's decision:

- **Medical situation**. Certain pre-existing diseases and disorders (e.g. blood clots, alcoholism, kidney problems, nutritional disorders) may cause complications during the operation or may even be aggravated by the operation itself.
- **Nutritional history**. One of the most important parameters is the person's ability to follow the diet: the nutritional history and the results obtained with diets followed in the past are evaluated.

The go-ahead for the operation is given only if other attempts have failed.

- **Psychological evaluation**. Undergoing bariatric surgery requires a balanced psychological condition: disorders such as anxiety, depression or post-traumatic stress can greatly frustrate the benefits of the surgical option.
- **Motivational evaluation**. Motivation is very important: the medical team must ensure that the person is able to radically change their lifestyle and adhere to a strict dietary plan.
- **Age and possible pathologies**. Usually it is considered that bariatric surgery is not advisable at a late age, as well as before the age of 18. Ideal candidates are patients between 18 and 65 years of age with third degree obesity (BMI over 30).

CHAPTER 3 - FOUR TYPES OF DIET TO FOLLOW AFTER SURGERY

A patient who has undergone bariatric surgery loses normal appetite for the first six weeks or so after surgery. Dietologists prescribe special light diets to meet the nutritional needs of the patient. A quality diet ensures proper healing and nutrition.

Recipes for patients undergoing bariatric surgery are available from dieticians and health specialists. Almost all these recipes contain a large amount of protein, which is essential for tissue growth and repair. Protein-rich foods are lower in calories and can therefore help maintain weight loss. The amount of protein needed should be calculated with a dietician. Foods rich in fat are best avoided as they can cause dumping syndrome and complicate the healing process. In addition to fat, sugar should also be avoided since it is difficult to digest. Recipes for patients undergoing bariatric surgery usually supplement sugar with honey. The amount of food is kept low to avoid digestive problems.

The food Pyramid after Bariatric Surgery

Every obesity surgery (bariatric surgery) - to satisfy every objective - must always be supported by a correct diet, which for many subjects is all to learn, or rather re-learn.

On the one hand, bariatric surgery, both restrictive and malabsorption, determines in the person an early sense of satiety and this leads to reduce quantities and eat less, on the other hand, after surgery the patient must learn to cooperate and eat properly. It's a bit like being weaned for the second time and not for everyone it's an easy situation even if in preliminary visits we talk a lot about it with our patients.

People who have undergone bariatric surgery (and often those close to them) need to change their eating habits, to be informed and know the various nutrients, to be able to choose the right foods and to be able to adhere to a new balanced diet even in the long term in a more conscious way, something they have not done for many years, also associating a physical activity program, perhaps starting from scratch because until then they have lived in a completely sedentary way.

The post-bariatric food pyramid is a slightly different instrument from the "classic" one because it has been studied ad hoc for patients who have been operated on with bariatric or metabolic surgery. It is a simple but very useful and practical tool, easy to consult for the patient.

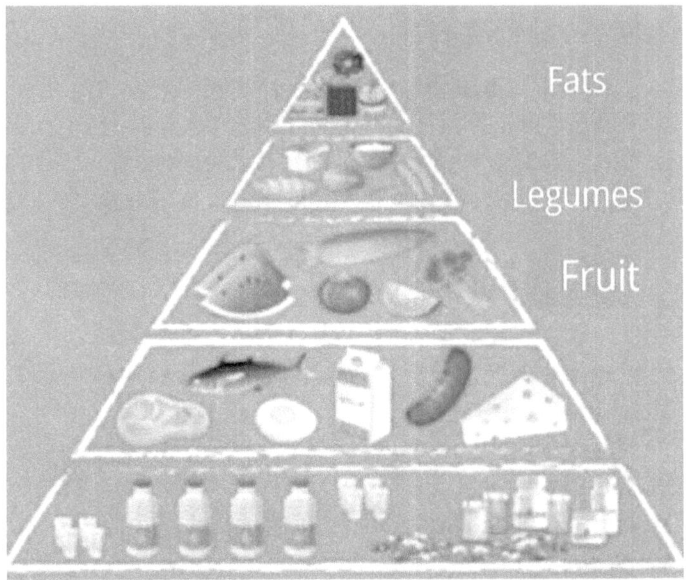

At the base of the pyramid, then on the first floor are visible the 'good habits' that the operated patient must adopt almost immediately: exercise daily, drink at least 1.5 litres of water per day, always chew carefully and take mineral supplements and vitamins as prescribed.

At the second level - unlike the traditional food pyramid - we do not have carbohydrates, but we have proteins. Why? Because the weight loss that patients undergo in the post-bariatric phase is considerable and very fast, it is not necessarily that you can only lose fat mass, more often you inevitably also lose lean mass, so to try to preserve lean mass patients must strictly try to implement the consumption of protein, which is not easy. Having this simple and visual tool helps the patient to remember that at least one of the main meals must be based on protein: only meat, only fish, only eggs, only cheese. Neither carbohydrates nor vegetables are provided as a side dish.

On the third level we have fruit and vegetables for the valuable intake of fibre, vitamins and minerals. At the penultimate level there are carbohydrates and at the apex, foods to be limited to the maximum: carbonated drinks, sweets and fatty condiments.

Liquid Diet

During the first period after the operation it is inevitable to follow a liquid diet, and then switch to a semi-liquid type of diet (with baby food, soft foods, creams and finely chopped ingredients). Subsequently, solid foods are gradually integrated, preferring digestible foods and paying attention to seasonings.

During the liquid diet the main dishes that can be consumed are the following:

- Semolina (very liquid)
- Filtered vegetable meat broth
- Vegetable broth milkshake (very liquid)
- Homogenized meat and fruit
- Milk (according to individual tolerance)
- Yogurt (preferably white without pieces)
- Biscuits for infants or buckets (dissolved in milk or tea)
- Fruit Juice

How to make homemade baby food

Homogenized Vegetable

First, prepare the vegetable broth that is the basis of all homogenized products. Take a carrot, a potato, a zucchini and some celery and dip everything in a litre of water, without adding salt. Boil for about an hour, until the water has halved. You can also use other vegetables for the broth, introducing them from week to week, such as artichokes, spinach, chard and everything your paediatrician will recommend.

Get all the utensils and small appliances that can serve you, such as mashers, blenders, or good homogenizers that you can easily find on the market at a very low cost.

The vegetable homogenizer is prepared by blending (or homogenizing) all the vegetables used to prepare the vegetable broth. When you blend them, add a little stock to mix them. At the end, add a drizzle of extra-virgin olive oil and perhaps some pastina or weaning cream. If you want to freeze the broth, you can use the ice cubes and put them in the freezer for about three months. If stored in the refrigerator, consume within 24 hours.

Homogenised meat

For the homogenized meat, be it chicken, beef, turkey, rabbit, choose parts that are non-fat, bone and cartilage free. Cook preferably with steam cooking that keeps the nutritional properties intact and greatly softens the meat. Use a steamer or a basket for steaming. When cooked, put the pieces of meat (cut small) in the homogenizer or blender, add the vegetables from the broth, about 100 ml of vegetable broth and a drizzle of extra virgin olive oil; then blend everything until you get a smooth cream.

Homogenized fish

The fish homogeniser follows the same procedure as the meat homogeniser. The most suitable fish are surely the cod, hake, sole; then add, month by month, other varieties according to the indications of the paediatrician. Clean the fish, steam it and then blend it in a blender with the vegetables that you need to prepare the broth.

Homogenized fruit

Fruit homogenisation requires the use of only two fruits, at least at the beginning of weaning, namely pear and apple. Take the chosen fruit (or both) and after having peeled it and removed the core, cut it into small pieces and steam it for about 10 minutes, until softened. After that, blend with a blender. The homogenizer is ready, and you can add milk or rice cream.

Homogenized meat, vegetables and fish

If you want to freeze the homogenized meat, vegetables and fish, pour them in vacuum-packed jars: in the freezer they last no longer than 6 months, in the fridge instead 24 hours. Fruit baby foods stored in the fridge should be consumed within 24 hours. For freezing, follow the advice of your doctor, who will tell you which fruit can be frozen, and which cannot.

FRUIT MILKSHAKE AND YOGHURT

Ingredients:

- 1 handful of blueberries
- 125 g low-fat white yoghurt
- milk (50 ml)
- 1 tablespoon of honey
- Ice

CARROT AND GREEN APPLE MILKSHAKE

Ingredients:

- 150 g carrots
- 2 green apples (Granny Smith)
- 1 lemon

Peel the apples and peel the carrots, then cut them into chunks. Put them in a blender and add the lemon juice. Blend for a few seconds. Pour into a tall glass and drink.

KIWI MILKSHAKE

Ingredients:

- 200 g of kiwi
- 2 tablespoons of low-fat yoghurt
- ½ glass of low-fat milk

Peel the kiwis and cut them into chunks. Put them in the blender with the milk and yogurt, blend them for a few moments. Pour into a glass and consume now.

ORANGE JUICE CENTRIFUGE

Ingredients:

- 1 glass of carrot juice
- ¼ glass of orange juice
- Grated peel of ½ orange
- 6 mint leaves
- A pinch of black pepper

Mix the juices in a carafe, add 4 mint leaves, orange peel, salt and pepper; put in the fridge for an hour and enjoy with ice cubes.

COURGETTE CENTRIFUGE

Ingredients:

- 2 small zucchinis
- 1 carrot
- 3 slices of cucumber
- 1 celery stalk
- ¼ golden apple
- A little piece of ginger
- A pinch of pepper

Wash the vegetables and peel the apple. Put everything into the centrifuge and run it until the juice is obtained; season the centrifuged mixture with chopped ginger, salt and pepper.

Semi-liquid Diet

Main dishes:

- Vegetable pastes
- Rice cream
- Very small pasta or milkshake
- Well-cooked minced meat and milkshakes
- Cooked or raw ham minced (without visible fat)

-   Soft low-fat cheeses (ricotta, flakes of milk)
-   Potato puree
-   Milk and fruit milkshakes, peeled and deprived of any seeds

MILD VEGETABLE PUREE

Ingredients for 4 people

-   1 kg mixed vegetables
-   2 decilitre whole milk
-   salt
-   extra virgin olive oil

Preparation of the past of delicate vegetables

1) Clean mixed vegetables (celery, carrots, peas, onions, potatoes, spinach, zucchini). Wash and cut into not too big chunks.

2) Cook the vegetables. Boil the vegetables in a pot with salted water and a little extra virgin olive oil. When the pieces are cooked, drain them without throwing away the cooking water.

3) Pass the vegetables to the mixer or vegetable masher. If the mixture is too thick, add a little of the cooking water. Salt rule.

4) To soften the taste of the vegetable mash, let it thicken slightly over high heat, then incorporate the hot milk and continue cooking for another 5 minutes.

5) Immediately distribute the delicate vegetable puree in the soup plates; before serving, garnish the surface with a round of warm milk.

FENNEL SAUCE WITH ANCHOVY RAGOUT

Ingredients for 4 people

-   pepper
-   1 spring onion
-   chili powder
-   extra virgin olive oil
-   2 tomatoes
-   salt

- 700 grams fennel
- 700 grams Sicilian or male anchovies or anchovies

1) To prepare the recipe for the fennel sauce with anchovy ragout, start washing the fennel, dry them, cut them into slices and put them in a steaming basket placed in a pot with a litre of fragrant water. Cook for about 35-40 minutes, then blend with 2 dl of cooking water, salt, pepper and keep them warm.

2) Wash the tomatoes, dry them and dice them. Slice the spring onion and let it flavour for a minute in a pan with 3 tablespoons of oil and a generous pinch of chilli pepper. Place the diced tomatoes and cook for another 5 minutes over high heat, then add the anchovies. Cook them for 10 minutes, always over high heat, add salt and stir, trying not to undone them too much.

3) Place the fennel cream prepared in 4 bowls, spread the anchovy sauce on top in the same quantity and serve immediately.

CREAM OF POTATOES AND NEW LEEKS

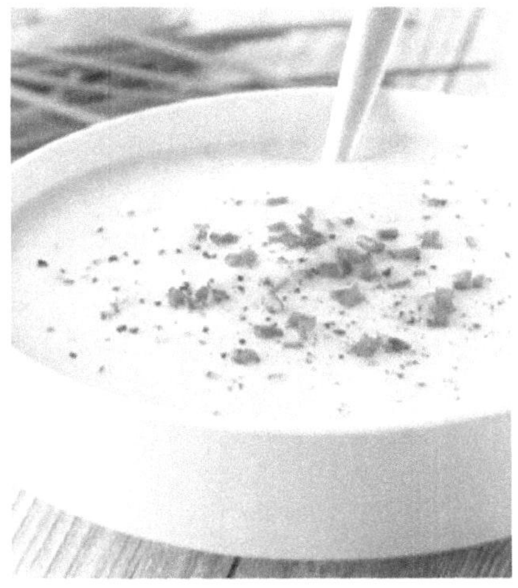

Ingredients for 4 people

- 50 grams butter
- 3 decilitres whole milk
- 60 grams smoked bacon or bacon

- 500 grams potato
- 200 grams shrimp tail
- vegetable stock
- 2 leeks
- salt
- extra virgin olive oil
- 1 tablespoon chives
- 6 pumpkin flowers
- Pepper

1) Start preparing the potato cream recipe by peeling the potatoes. Wash them and cut them into pieces. Also clean the leeks, wash them and slice them. Leave these two ingredients to flavour in a saucepan with butter.

2) Add the milk to the potatoes and leeks, cover the casserole and continue cooking for 20 minutes. If necessary, add a ladle of hot broth.

3) Adjust salt and pepper and turn off the heat. Blend to form a homogeneous cream and let it cool.

4) Wrap the shrimps with slices of bacon and let them brown for a few seconds in a little oil.

5) Spread the cream on the bottom of the plates.

6) Serve the cream of potatoes and leeks garnished with the shrimps and chives.

CREAM OF COURGETTES WITH SQUIDS

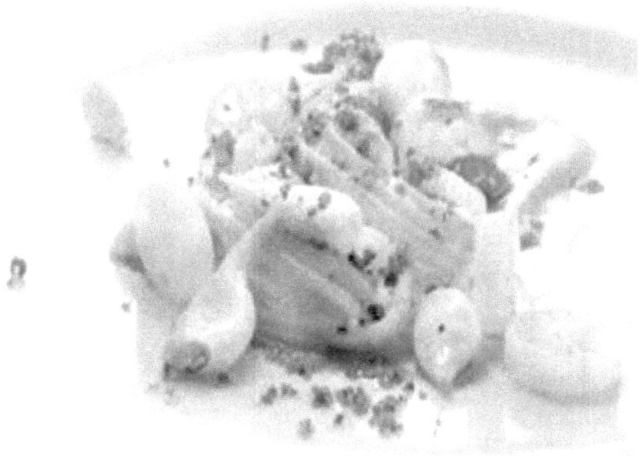

Ingredients for 6 people

- extra virgin olive oil
- 10 shrimp tails
- 1.5 litre vegetable stock
- black pepper grains
- 1-kilogram zucchini
- 300 grams tattler
- salt
- 150 grams potatoes
- 1 leek

1) To prepare the zucchini cream recipe, wash the zucchini and remove the ends. Remove the leek from the roots, the outer part and the green leaves. Peel also the potato and reduce everything to chunks.

2) Bring the broth to the boil and add the vegetables. Let them cook covered over medium heat for 20 minutes.

3) Remove the intestinal thread from the shrimp tails and boil them in boiling salted water for one minute. Drain them and let them cool before removing the carapace. Cut them in half lengthwise and then reduce them to chunks. Rinse the squids and cut the bags into strips.

4) Heat 2 tablespoons of oil in a non-stick pan and, as soon as it is hot, add the strips of squid that will accompany the cream of zucchini. Cook for a minute stirring frequently and, if necessary, add a pinch of salt.

LENTIL AND VEGETABLE SOUP

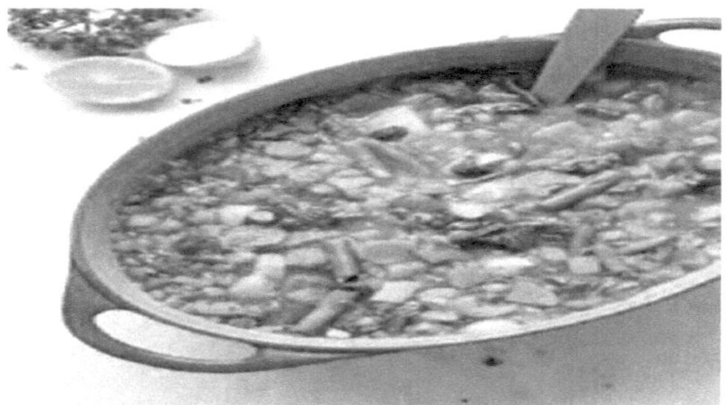

Lentil soup with spring vegetables is a nutritious and tasty first course, enriched with seasonal vegetables such as chard and zucchini and flavoured with sage leaves.

Ingredients:

- 200 grams of dried lentils
- 350 grams of chard
- 1 potato
- 2 zucchini
- 1 carrot
- 1 coppered tomato
- 3-4 sage leaves
- pecorino
- extra virgin olive oil
- salt
- pepper

Procedure

Wash and cut the vegetables: the carrots into rounds, the potatoes and zucchini into chunks, the tomato first into slices and then into cubes.

Remove the chard from the ribs and leathery parts and cut them into strips.

Rinse the lentils and pour them into an earthenware pan with the vegetables, cover with water and cook for about 40 minutes, until both vegetables and lentils have softened.

Add the chopped sage leaves, season with salt and pepper and cook for a few more minutes.

Seasoned with a drizzle of extra virgin olive oil and a sprinkling of pecorino cheese.

VELVETY PUMPKIN SOUP

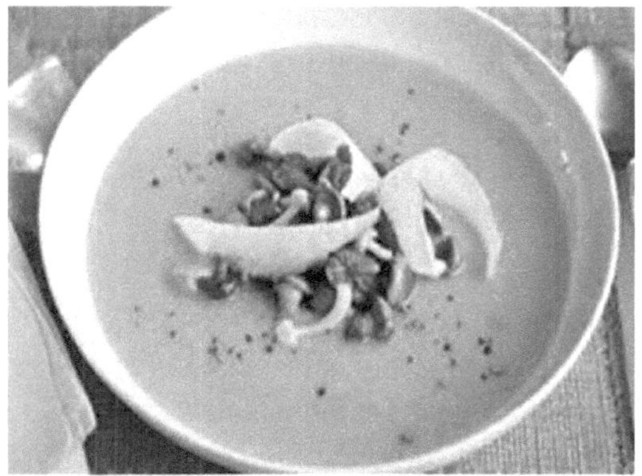

Ingredients for 4 people

-   450 grams pumpkin
-   50 grams almond flour
-   50 grams butter
-   10 grams sugar
-   2 untreated oranges
-   2 yolks
-   8 decilitres vegetable stock
-   1 tablespoon white vinegar
-   1 tuft coriander
-   cinnamon powder
-   grated Parmesan cheese
-   toasts
-   salt
-   pepper

Preparation of the pumpkin velveteen

1) First of all, to prepare the velvet, wash the pumpkin thoroughly, remove the seeds and obtain from the edge of the pumpkin some thin slices with the peel to keep aside.

2) Remove the remaining pumpkin skin, cut the flesh into pieces, collect them in a saucepan and cover them completely with the hot broth, put them on the stove and bring everything to the boil. Let it simmer for 12-15 minutes, stirring occasionally with a wooden spoon, until the pumpkin starts to melt.

3) At this point, first blend the pumpkin with a mixer. Then take a large non-stick pan and heat 30 g of butter. Add and toast the almond flour, add also the pumpkin cream and mix to obtain a thick and lump-free pumpkin creamy soup

4) Continue the recipe for pumpkin velveteen by heating the velveteen obtained and, if it is too thick, dilute it with a ladleful of hot broth.

5) Wash the oranges and grate one teaspoon of the peel. Squeeze the oranges and add the juice to the velveteen. Heat it again and, a moment before removing it from the heat, add the two yolks and stir immediately vigorously. At this point rule of salt and pepper, also incorporate the orange peel kept aside and turn it off.

6) Take a small non-stick pan and melt the remaining butter with 10 g of sugar and vinegar. When the sugar is amber, caramelize the pumpkin slices kept aside in the pan for about 1 minute.

7) Distribute the velvet obtained in 4 soup plates, garnish with the caramelized pumpkin slices and coriander. Sprinkle with a pinch of cinnamon and serve the velvety pumpkin soup with grated Parmesan cheese and bread croutons.

AUBERGINE CREAM WITH CROUTONS

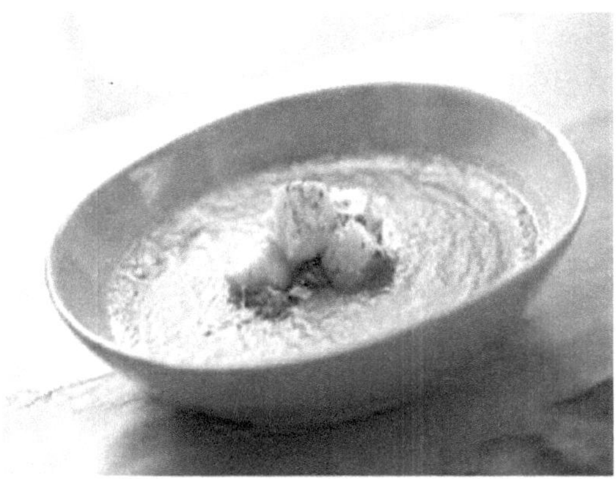

Ingredients for 4 people

- 1.5 kg eggplant
- chili pepper
- 250 grams whole yoghurt
- 0.5 clove garlic
- 1 fresh marjoram sprig
- 2 slices of bread
- 1 teaspoon tomato paste
- extra virgin olive oil
- salt

How to prepare aubergine cream with croutons

1) Wash and dry the aubergines by removing the ends and peel them with a potato peeler, keeping 1/4 of the skin of an aubergine aside. Cut the pulp into cubes and place them on a baking tray covered with greaseproof paper. Add a pinch of salt and a drizzle of extra virgin olive oil and bake at 180° for about 30 minutes. Check the cooking and stir from time to time.

2) Take the baking pan out of the oven, pass the eggplant pulp together with the tomato paste to the mixer, incorporate the yoghurt into the cream thus obtained, mix. Chop the peeled garlic and marjoram leaves and add a little of this chopped mixture to the mixture.

3) Brush the slices of bread with oil and cut them into slices, then toast them in a non-stick pan until golden brown. In the meantime, heat the oil and,

when it is well hot, dip the julienne-cut eggplant peel into it. Drain with a perforated ladle and remove the excess oil by placing it on a plate lined with absorbent paper.

4) Serve the eggplant cream with croutons at the beginning of the meal, together with the crispy eggplant skin and, if desired, with a pinch of chilli pepper.

VELVETY PUMPKIN AND POTATO SOUP WITH CHESTNUTS

Ingredients for 6 people

- pepper
- 200 grams pumpkin
- 1 bay leaf
- 1.2 decilitre vegetable stock
- 8 chestnut
- 2 tablespoons olive oil
- 2 potato
- salt
- 1 onion
- 1/2 tablespoon apple vinegar
- new oil

How to make pumpkin and potato velvet with chestnuts

1) To make the recipe for pumpkin and potato velvet with chestnuts, first cut 2 potatoes, 200 g pumpkin and 6 peeled chestnuts into small cubes; add a bay leaf, 1.2 dl vegetable stock and bring to the boil. Fry one onion with 2 tablespoons of oil, salt, sprinkle it with half a tablespoon of apple vinegar; let it evaporate, then caramelize the onion over low heat and add it to the broth the last 5 minutes of cooking.

2) Blend the vegetables and add salt and pepper. Finely slice 2 more chestnuts and dry them in the oven at 80°C for 5 minutes. Pour the velvety pumpkin and potato soup into the bowls, season with new Tuscan olive oil and sprinkle with dried chestnuts.

VELVETY SOUP WITH CELERY AND CABBAGE

Ingredients for 6 people

- pepper
- 2 litre vegetable stock
- 1 garlic clove
- 400 grams chestnut
- 40 grams grain
- extra virgin olive oil
- 6 celery
- 2 slices celeriac (celeriac of Verona)
- 1 onion
- 2 cabbage leaves
- croutons

Preparation of the velveteen with celery and cabbage

1) To cook the velvety recipe with celery and cabbage, sauté the chopped onion together with 2 tablespoons of oil in a large saucepan; when it becomes transparent, add 5 sliced celery ribs and the cabbage cut into strips.

2) Let the vegetables sauté for a short time, add the chestnuts, stir for a couple of minutes and pour in the broth; boil for 30 minutes. Turn off the heat, put the soup in the mixer glass and blend until the consistency becomes homogeneous.

3) In the meantime, sauté the sliced garlic in a pan with 2 tablespoons of oil, add the diced celery from Verona and the finely sliced celery rib.

4) Tie the velveteen together with the grated grana cheese if you like, put it on the plates and sprinkle it with the fried celery. Add a drizzle of raw oil and pepper to taste and accompany with some bread croutons baked in the oven to be served separately.

PEAR AND GINGER JAM

Ingredients:

- 1kg pears
- 450 gr of sugar
- Half lemon juices
- 1 piece of ginger

Put the peeled and chopped pears in a pot with the sugar, lemon juice and the peeled and grated ginger. Boil for about half an hour, remove the foam that forms on the surface with a skimmer. With an immersion blender blend everything and bring it back to the fire. Try the saucer, i.e. put a spoonful of jam on the saucer if it has the consistency you like it will be ready.

RED PUMPKIN WITH BALSAMIC VINEGAR

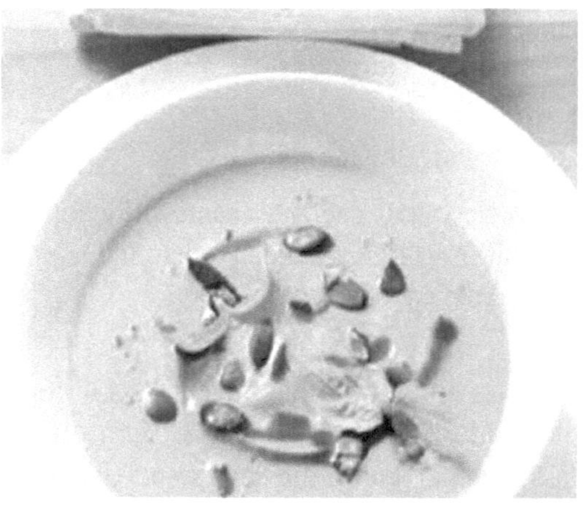

Ingredients:

- 1kg of red pumpkin
- 2 large onions
- 2 cloves of garlic
- 1/2 glass of balsamic vinegar
- Extra virgin olive oil
- Hello and pepper

Clean the pumpkin, cut into cubes and place in a bowl, add the sliced onions, garlic (whole or cut small), 2 tablespoons of evo oil, balsamic vinegar, salt and pepper. Stir to give flavour and pour everything into a baking tray. Bake at 200° ventilated combined with grill on top. The pumpkin needs at least 45 minutes to cook, you must stir occasionally and check the cooking. Ready, you'll discover what a smell and goodness!

Soft Diet

Main dishes:

- Soft polenta
- Thicker vegetable and rice cream pastes
- Small pastry seasoned with tomato sauce or oil and parmesan cheese
- Steamed fish
- Boiled or steamed chicken or turkey
- Boiled vegetables with less fibre content (carrots, zucchini, herbs)
- Crushed or grated fruit (apple, banana)

BOILED TURKEY

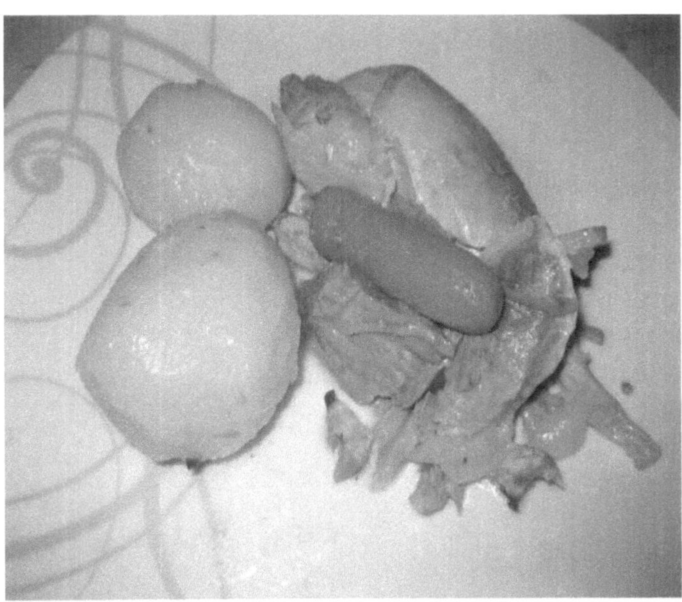

Ingredients:

- 2 turkey spindles
- 4 potatoes
- 4 carrots

- 1 golden onion
- 1 tomato
- salt
- parsley

Procedure:

First if you have bones of any kind of meat place them in a pot, cover them with water and let them cook for an hour on medium heat. At this point filter the remaining stock and put it back into the pot. Peel the potatoes and carrots and add them to the broth, cutting the carrots in half. Also add the onion cut into 4 and the peeled and chopped tomatoes.

Finally add the spindles, a tuft of parsley, salt and cover with water. When it starts to boil, cook it for 1 hour and a half until the meat is tender. At this point you can use the broth to accompany some tagliolini or tortelli as you like.

STEAMED CHICKEN

Ingredients

- 600 gr chicken breast
- 3 shallots
- 1 celery ribbed (stalk)
- 1 carrot
- 2 dl vegetable stock
- 2 tablespoons mustard beans
- 2 tablespoons soy sauce
- 1 teaspoon tomato paste
- 1 teaspoon curry
- 1 bunch of parsley
- 1 bay leaf
- chives
- extra virgin olive oil
- salt

The steamed chicken steak is a second course of super light white meat but rich in taste. Learn how to prepare it at home by following the instructions in this easy step-by-step recipe, you'll enjoy a nutritious dish with only 224 calories per serving.

As an alternative to the 2 sauces that we present here you can accompany the course with a diced tomato enriched with arugula leaves, flakes of Parmesan cheese and a few drops of balsamic vinegar. Or you can prepare a yoghurt sauce by mixing 1 jar of yoghurt with 1 piece of peeled and grated ginger root, 1 zucchini and 1 carrot chopped with the white part of 1 spring onion, 1 pinch of salt and chili pepper and some chopped mint leaves.

Steam the chicken. Cut the celery and carrot into chunks, put them in the saucepan with the parsley stalks and the bay leaf. Place the steaming basket on top and pour in enough water to touch the bottom of the basket. Transfer the chicken fillets, cover and cook over low heat for 15-20 minutes after boiling.

Prepare the first sauce. Cut the shallots, skin them and cut them into very thin slices. Put them in a saucepan with the curry, 1 pinch of salt and 2 tablespoons of water, cover and cook over low heat for 3-4 minutes. Add the tomato paste, dilute with the broth, stir to amalgamate and continue cooking over a covered pot for about 10-15 minutes.

Prepare the second raw sauce. Rinse the chives under a jet of cold running water, dry it and cut it with scissors. Combine it in a bowl with chopped parsley leaves, mustard, soy sauce and 2 tablespoons of extra virgin olive oil, then emulsify the ingredients, beating them vigorously with a whisk or fork.

Use the meat and serve it at the table. Let the chicken breast cool down, cut it into thin slices, horizontally, and bring to the table the steamed chicken cut with the two accompanying sauces.

RICE CREAM

The cream of rice is very simple and quick to prepare. An ancient recipe prepared all over the world that adults and children alike like for its simplicity and its soft and creamy taste. A perfect dessert for a quick snack or for a moment of relaxation in company. It is ideal if accompanied by chocolate chips, cinnamon or fresh fruit, the result is guaranteed!

How to prepare the cream of rice

To prepare the rice cream, start by pouring the milk into a pan, add a stick of cinnamon and some lemon or orange peel to flavour it and leave to boil.

1) Rinse the rice so that it loses some of its floury consistency. Pour the rice and sugar into the boiling milk, stirring with a whisk to prevent lumps from forming.

2) Cook for about 10 minutes taking care that the rice does not stick to the bottom of the pan and at the same time absorb the milk while cooking. When your cream is thick and creamy, remove from the heat, let it rest for a few minutes and finally pour the mixture into single-portion moulds.

3), cover with transparent film and leave to rest in the fridge for about 2 hours. Serve with a sprinkling of cinnamon, cocoa or fresh fruit. Decorate with a mint leaf.

SOFT POLENTA

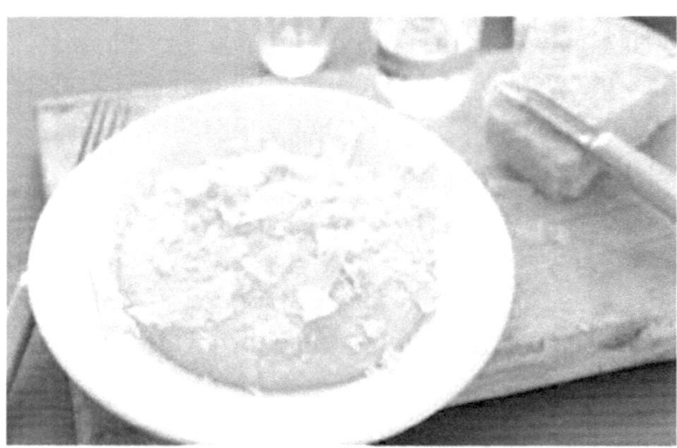

Ingredients for 4 people:

- 250 g of flour for polenta
- 1/2 litre milk
- 1/2 litre water
- a knob of butter
- salt.

Preparation

Mix the polenta flour with the water and milk. Cook it for 45/60 minutes (the cooking time depends on the flour you buy, look on the package) always stirring first with a whisk to avoid the formation of lumps then use a wooden ladle.

At the end of cooking over a low heat add the butter.

Serve immediately.

GENOESE ZUCCHINI PESTO

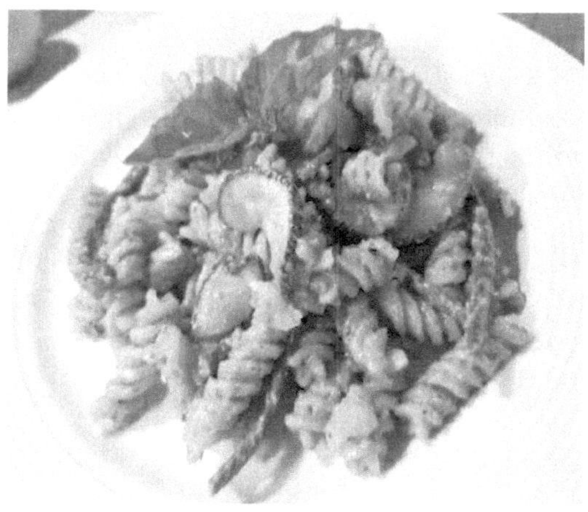

Ingredients:

For the pesto:

- 3 Genoese zucchini
- 100 gr of almonds
- 2 cloves of garlic
- 1 bunch of basil
- 2 tablespoons of grated Parmesan cheese
- 2 tablespoons of grated pecorino romano cheese
- Extra virgin olive oil 8/10 spoons
- Salt and pepper

For the pasta:

(4 people)

- 400 gr of fusilli
- 1 Genoese courgette
- 1 large potato

- 15 green beans
- Frying oil
- salt

Prepare the pesto: grate the zucchini with the whole skin and put them in a colander for about half an hour. Clean and dry the basil.

In the meantime, cut the zucchini into rounds for the pasta, fry and salt.

After the zucchini have lost their water, prepare the pesto. In a mixer put the garlic, almonds and a few tablespoons of evo oil. Blend everything. Then add the zucchini and basil, add a few more tablespoons of evo oil and blend again. Finally put the grated cheese, taste and adjust the salt and if you like you can add a little pepper or chilli pepper. The pesto is ready!

For the pasta: in the pot where to cook the pasta, put the chopped potatoes and green beans. When the water boils add the fusilli and salt. Cook, drain and put back into the pot. Add the zucchini pesto, mix well, plate and garnish each portion with the zucchini previously fried. Ready and delicious!

RICE WITH COOKED

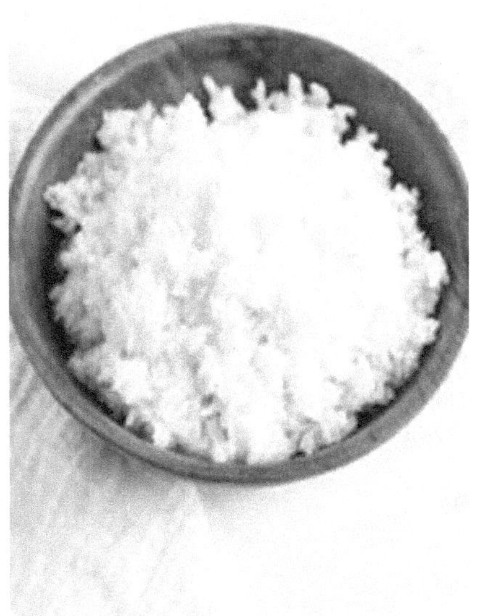

Ingredients:

- 20 gr of rice
- 30 gr of terracotta
- 2 teaspoons of parmesan cheese
- 1 teaspoon of butter...

Cook the rice in a saucepan with a small piece of dice. Cut the cooked ham into fine strips and add it to the rice. When cooked, turn off the stove and add butter and Parmesan cheese.

ZUCCHINI FLAN

Ingredients:

- oil
- 4 zucchini
- 1 clove of garlic
- 100 ml béchamel
- 2 eggs

- 4 tablespoons of parmesan cheese
- 1 roll of puff pastry
- 2 goat cheeses
- salt

Preparation:

Wash and cut the courgettes and then fry them in a knob of butter, soften them over a low heat, add salt and pepper and when they are cooked, transfer them to a bowl and blend them. Add the béchamel sauce, eggs, Parmesan cheese, salt and pepper and mix. Butter a plum cake mould, then pour the mixture and bake at 180° for 40'. Remove from the oven, cover with the goat cheese and a rectangle of pastry and bake again for another 15'-20' in a ventilated oven. Remove from the oven, allow to cool for a few minutes and place the flan on a serving plate.

FENNEL AU GRATIN WITH BACON

Ingredients:

- 2 fennel
- three tablespoons of grated Parmesan cheese
- 2 slices of speck half a centimetre high
- 250 ml béchamel

Preparation:

Wash and slice the fennel and then blanch them in boiling salted water for a few minutes. Drain them and let them cool. In the meantime, take the two slices of speck deprived of the fat and pepper and chop them in the mixer. Put all the other ingredients together in a bowl and mix them with the chopped speck.

Pour everything into an ovenproof dish lined with baking paper, add a sprinkling of grain and put in the oven until the crust forms. Turn off the oven and let the fennel cool down and serve warm.

SWEET AND SOUR PEPPERS WITH OLIVES AND MINT

Ingredients:

- 4 red peppers
- 200 gr of pitted olives
- 2 big onions
- 15 mint leaves
- 1 glass of tomato sauce
- 1 glass of white vinegar
- 1 glass of sugar
- 3 tablespoons of extra virgin olive oil
- Salt and pepper

Put the peppers on a baking tray and bake at 200 °, turn them from time to time. As soon as they are cooked, let them cool and then skin them and cut them into pieces. Fry the sliced onions in a pan, add the tomato sauce and cook them. As soon as the onions are cooked, add the vinegar and sugar, continue to cook until they have thickened a bit. Add the olives. Taste the sweet and sour and adjust if necessary, with the sugar. Add salt and pepper to taste. Finally, add the mint leaves. Ready to taste!

TUNA MEATLOAF

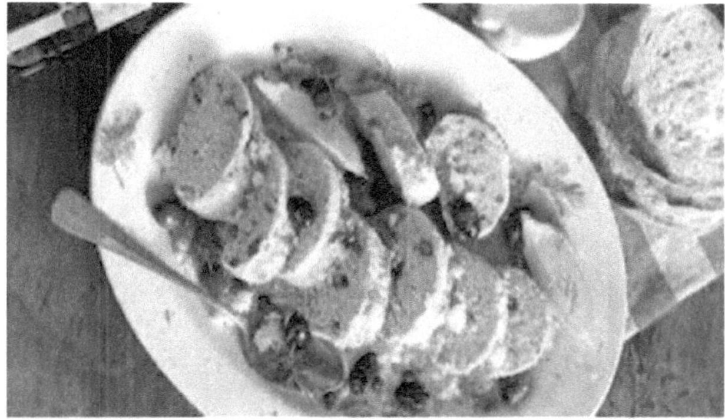

Ingredients:

- 1 potato
- 2 cans of tuna 180 gr
- 1 egg
- 2 tablespoons of parmesan cheese

- 1 tablespoon parsley
- 2 tablespoons of breadcrumbs or two slices of finely chopped breadcrumbs
- 1 tablespoon of mixed fried food
- 2 tablespoons of white wine
- salt

Boil the potato then crush it with a coarse fork, then drain the tuna well and chop it. Then add all the other ingredients, mix them all together until you get a homogeneous mixture. Give the mixture the classic meatloaf shape and wrap it with baking paper like a candy, put it in an oven dish and bake it in the oven for about thirty minutes until it reaches an intense golden colour.

Turn off the oven and leave the door slightly open. Once lukewarm, cut it into slices of about one centimetre and serve it with the side dish you prefer.

AUBERGINE SLICES

Ingredients

For the sfincione sauce:

- 4 onions
- 1 kg of peeled tomatoes
- 6 anchovy fillets in oil
- Fresh Oregano
- Extra virgin olive oil
- 3 aubergines
- 150 gr of grated semi-seasoned caciocavallo cheese
- 100 gr of semi-seasoned caciocavallo cheese
- 150 gr of breadcrumbs
- Anchovies in oil
- Extra virgin olive oil

Wash and cut the aubergines, roast them. At the same time prepare the dressing for the sfincione sauce. In a pot put the thinly sliced onions, the anchovies with a few tablespoons of evo oil. Leave to cook over moderate heat, making sure that the onion does not burn, if necessary, add a little water. As soon as the onion is cooked, add the peeled sauce previously blended, leave to cook, season with salt and pepper and if necessary, add a little sugar. When the sauce is ready, add the oregano on a low flame.

Put some evo oil on the bottom and proceed in layers: first the roasted aubergines, then the sfincione sauce, a sprinkling of grated caciocavallo cheese and again aubergines, sauce and caciocavallo, make no more than three layers. For the last layer on top of the sauce and the caciocavallo, put the breadcrumbs previously seasoned with evo oil, add small pieces of cacio cavallo and small pieces of anchovy in oil and bake for about 10 minutes, as long as the surface is well browned. The aubergines a sfincione are now ready to taste!

RICOTTA AND TUNA MEATBALLS

Ingredients:

- 250 grams of ricotta cheese
- 160 gr of tuna in oil
- 2 eggs
- Breadcrumbs

Drain the oil from the tuna, put in the blender, blend together the ricotta cheese and eggs, blend again, add breadcrumbs just enough to have a soft dough neither too liquid nor too hard, a little 'salt then made the meatballs, pass them in the breadcrumbs and bake in the oven for about a quarter of an hour.

SPRING ROLLS

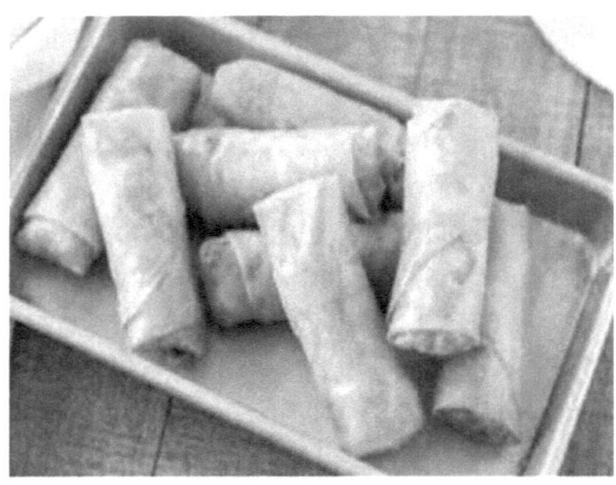

Ingredients:

- One or two packs of fillo pasta (depends on how many you want to make)
- 2/3 zucchini per size
- 2/3 carrots
- if you also want 1 eggplant
- 1 shallot or spring onion
- Soy sauce
- salt
- chili pepper
- Shrimps or chicken breast

Cut the vegetables into thin strips, heat a non-stick pot well and throw out the vegetables, adjust with soy sauce and a little (I said a little) water or white wine.

When the vegetables are well withered add either the shrimps in small pieces or a slice of grilled chicken breast in small pieces (you can of course also make only vegetables).

Prepare in a cup a spoon or two of oil, chilli pepper and water and emulsify well, this will be used to brush the pasta fillo both to close and out.

Make the rolls and bake in the oven at 200 ° C for 15 minutes, even less: it depends on the oven you see when you colour the dough since inside are already cooked).

RADICCHIO AND GOAT'S MILK RISOTTO

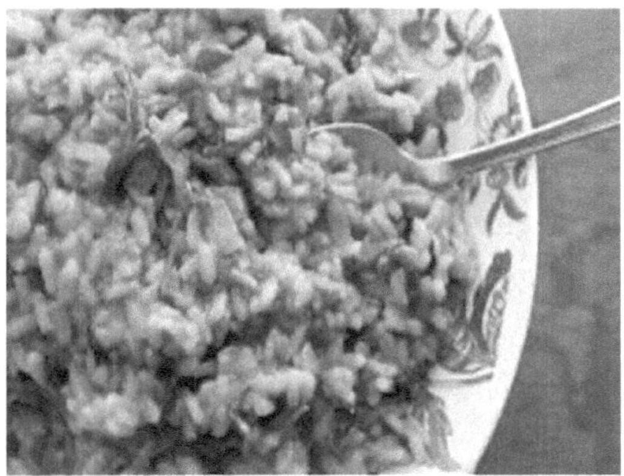

Ingredients:

-   40 gr rice
-   1 radicchio leaf
-   Vegetable broth
-   Half goat
-   Half red onion

Procedure:

In a pan brown some onion with half a glass of white wine, apart from preparing a vegetable broth with 1 carrot 1 zucchini half an onion. Toast the rice and cook gradually by putting a ladleful of broth and bring to cooking. After 10 minutes, put the radicchio cut into strips, at the end of cooking add the goat's half. The broth with the vegetables can be blended in the evening. If you add a little oil and 1 tablespoon grana cheese, you can use the mixture as a vegetable mash for the evening.

PIGEONFISH SALAD

Ingredients:

-   200 g boiled green beans
-   3 boiled potatoes al dente
-   300 g pigeonhole
-   lemon
-   oil

- basil
- salt and pepper

Dice the bumblebee and steam (or microwave) it for 10 minutes.

Cut the green beans into chunks and the potatoes into slices, mix them with the bumblebee and season with lemon juice, salt, pepper and some chopped basil leaves.

ZUCCHINI CARPACCIO

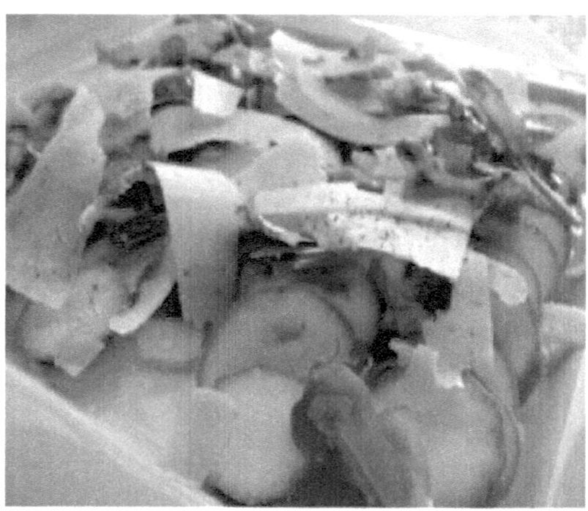

Ingredients:

- 4 tender zucchini
- 100 g of parmesan cheese flakes
- 1 lemon
- 1 bunch of parsley
- 1 bunch of basil
- Extra virgin olive oil
- Pepper
- salt

Wash and dry the zucchini, then trim them at the ends. Slice them lengthwise with a potato peeler, if you don't have one, use a very sharp knife.

Squeeze the lemon. Filter the juice, add the oil, a pinch of salt and emulsify to obtain a homogeneous sauce.

Coarsely chop the parsley and basil.

Now arrange the zucchini in a serving dish or, if you prefer, in a bowl. Make layers and pour on each layer a little sauce, parsley and basil, pepper and parmesan flakes.

Tips

The zucchini carpaccio can be eaten freshly made but if you prepare it a couple of hours earlier it will be tastier. The ideal would be to prepare this dish the night before, so that the zucchini can take the taste of marinating well.

Ideas and variations

Instead of basil, you can use chives or a very thinly sliced clove of garlic. Also, if it is to your taste, you can decorate the last layer of zucchini with capers and black olives.

LIGHT LENTIL AND TUNA MEATBALLS

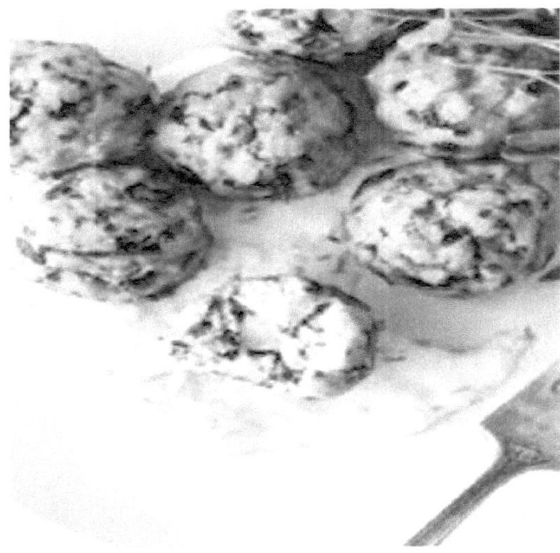

Ingredients for 20 meatballs:

- 240gr of canned lentils well drained
- a can of tuna natural 100gr
- half onion
- a clove of garlic
- an egg
- 2 tablespoons of grated Parmesan cheese
- 2 tablespoons of breadcrumbs
- salt and pepper

To prepare the lentil and tuna meatballs, all you must do is put all the ingredients in the mixer except the breadcrumbs, blend everything for a few seconds. Put the mixture in a bowl and add the breadcrumbs and mix well, after which leave in the fridge for about an hour. When the mixture is ready you can bake it in a non-stick pan or in the oven.

BAKED VEGETABLE PANCAKES

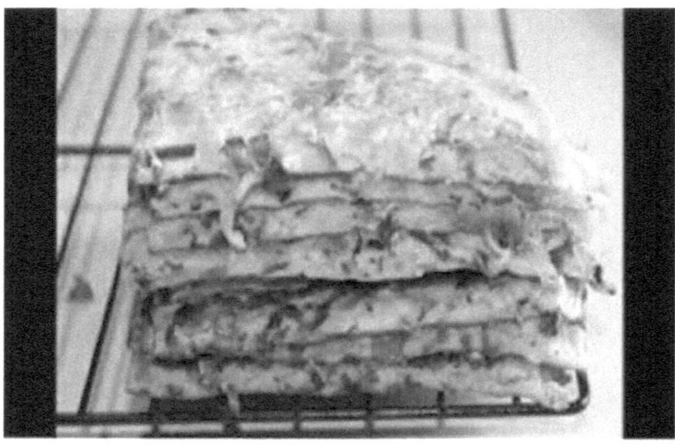

Ingredients

- 5 eggs
- 1 small-medium potato (100g)
- 1 small zucchini (240g)
- 1/2 small eggplant (80g)
- 1/2 red pepper (100g.)
- 1 medium red onion (110g)
- 1/2 box of peeled tomatoes
- 1 teaspoon of EVO oil

- salt and black pepper to taste
- oregano to taste

Turn the oven up to 180 degrees. Cut all the vegetables into small cubes and place them, with the peeled tomatoes, salt, pepper and oregano in a baking pan.

Cook for about 45 minutes, turning often. The vegetables should be tender. In case the tomato tends to pull too much, add a few tablespoons of water.

Once cooked, without turning off the oven, let it cool out of the oven while, in a very large bowl, beat the eggs.

Add the cooked vegetables to the eggs and divide the mixture into a 12-place muffin pan lightly greased with a spoonful of oil (or, if you prefer, using the paper cups of the right size).

Bake in the oven for 30/35 minutes until golden brown.

Once cooled, the pancakes can be frozen.

FLOURLESS PIZZA

A cauliflower-based mixture is used, and you can choose between two recipes.

It is not a dough prepared with alternative flours and gluten free, but a cauliflower-based mixture that is then seasoned to taste with tomato, mozzarella and much more, just like a real pizza.

This recipe is a "low calories" idea for those who are on a diet, but do not want to deprive themselves of the taste of a good pizza every now and then, but it is also a tasty and light alternative for those who are intolerant to flour and want to try something new.

There are two recipes for flourless pizza. One involves the use of whole eggs, and the other a chopped almond and egg white.

The consistency will obviously not be identical to that of a classic pizza prepared with a leavened dough base, but it will still be very crunchy, and the taste of cauliflower will not be too invasive.

After washing the cauliflower and removing the leaves and stem, dry it with kitchen paper and chop it very finely. It is important that it is well dry otherwise the mixture will not be crunchy.

If you use almonds, also chop them finely, or opt for those already reduced to flour.

Recipe with eggs

Chop very finely a washed cauliflower with the leaves removed and then add two beaten eggs and enough Parmesan cheese to reach a pasty consistency.

Season with a pinch of salt and place this mixture on a well-oiled baking tray by pressing it with your hands. Cook for 30 minutes at 150°.

Then season with tomato puree and mozzarella or as you prefer and cook for another 10 minutes.

Recipe with almonds

Chop also in this case a well washed and dried cauliflower with the leaves removed.

With the cauliflower finely chopped even 40 gr of almonds, a pinch of salt and dried oregano.

Add to this mixture an egg white and mix well.

proceed with the cooking as in the previous recipe.

SOYA SPAGHETTI

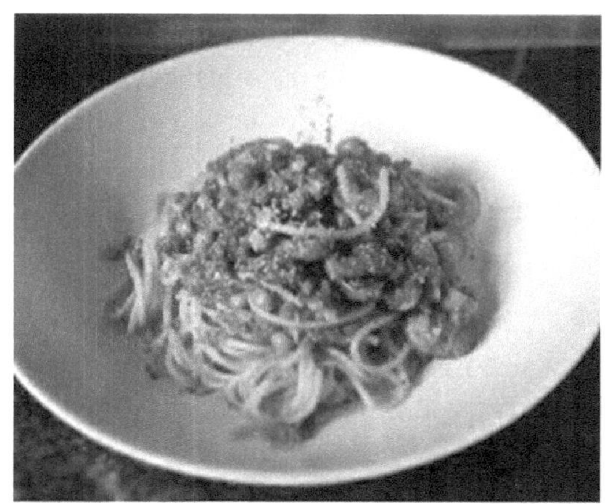

Soya spaghetti, typical of oriental cuisine, has now become an easy to find food on the Italian market, not only for its organoleptic properties, but also for its well-known healthy properties. Excellent source of protein and iron with low fat content, they are therefore a valid substitute for the common wheat pasta. If, once purchased, you are faced with the dilemma of how to prepare them and which is the seasoning that best enhances their quality and taste, continue reading: you will find instructions to prepare 5 condiments with which to taste the best soy spaghetti. You will discover that they are very versatile and can be enjoyed both as the classic pasta sauce and in salad and broth.

In tomato sauce

Let's start with a simple and healthy recipe: the classic tomato sauce, Italian style. In a non-stick pan, heat 2 tablespoons of olive oil over medium heat. Add 1 clove of sliced garlic, let it brown, then pour into the pan 500 gr of fresh tomatoes (pachino type) roughly cut or 400 gr of tomato pulp, adjust the salt and bring the sauce to a light boil, stirring occasionally. To give a Mediterranean touch to the sauce you can add a few black Kalamata or "taggiasca" olives cut into rounds, 1 chilli pepper and a pinch of oregano. Once drained the spaghetti, sauté them in tomato sauce and serve on the table, with a nice grated Parmesan or pecorino cheese.

Sautéed with vegetables

In a preheated wok, heat 2 tablespoons of olive oil, where you then wither 1 chopped shallot. Add 1/2 zucchini, 1/2 eggplant and 1/2 red pepper cut into cubes and leave to cook over a high flame, so that the vegetables remain crispy, being careful to stir frequently, so that they do not stick. After 15 minutes, add 1 handful of pine nuts. Then dip the cooked spaghetti al dente in the wok, add the seasoning for 1 minute and bring to the table.

Salad

Fresh solution that can be a one-size-fits-all. In a large bowl pour 2 tablespoons of soy sauce, 1 teaspoon of sugar, 2 tablespoons of seed oil, the juice of ½ lemon and a pinch of cumin. Mix well to emulsify the ingredients, add the cooked spaghetti, drained under cold water, crab meat or surimi, peeled shrimps sautéed or boiled and 1 teaspoon of finely chopped chives. Stir to amalgamate and enjoy. The salad is one of the dishes that best lends itself to personalization: try it also with the addition of edamame (soybeans), toasted soybeans, broccoli sprouts, sliced champignons and thin slices of chili pepper, to give a touch of colour. Alternatively, you can replace the fish with pan-fried or grilled chicken breast cut into strips.

Oriental soup

Noodles style, sweet-sour and slightly spicy taste. Cut 1 slice of beef into strips and marinate it in 1 tablespoon of soy sauce. Meanwhile, prepare the stock by melting ½ meat cube in 750 ml of water, to which add 1 tablespoon of soy sauce and 1 bunch of sliced herbs or chard. Bring to the boil and, after 4/5 minutes, add the beef strips and soy spaghetti cooked al dente and drained. Continue cooking for a couple of minutes, turn off the heat, add 1 tablespoon of chopped fresh parsley and the juice of 1 lime. Place in a bowl and serve the soup hot and steaming.

Flavourful seasoning

To finish, I propose a condiment with Asian smells: soy spaghetti with pork and vegetables. The flavour of soya with pork is attenuated by cabbage, in a rather tasty combination. Finely chopped 1 celery stalk and 1 spring onion. Transfer them to a pan, where you have previously withered 1 tablespoon of freshly chopped ginger with 1 tablespoon of oil. At this point you can add 200 gr of minced pork, 200 gr of cabbage cut into thin strips and sauté over high heat for 5 minutes, stirring continuously. Pour the spaghetti cooked in salted water, 1 tablespoon of soy sauce, add salt and pepper and let it season for 5 minutes. To give an oriental touch, decorate with a grated fresh ginger.

Soya spaghetti, especially if served with vegetable seasonings or in soup, make more than durum wheat, so remember to reduce the portions.

All the above ingredients yield for 2 servings.

LEAN PORK WITH TOMATO JAM

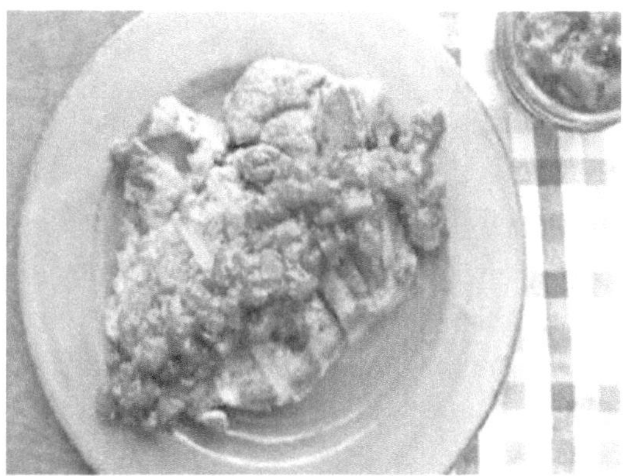

Ingredients

- Arista tied and harnessed with bacon 1 kg
- Salt up to
- Black pepper
- Garlic 2 cloves
- White wine 80 g
- Courgettes 500 g
- Water 30 g
- Thyme
- Extra virgin olive oil

For tomato jam

- Tomatoes 500 g
- Sugar 150 g
- Red onions ½
- White wine vinegar 50 g

- Salt up to
- Chilli powder ¼ teaspoon

Preparation

To make the pork arista with tomato jam first get an arista already tied up, dressed with bacon and splinted with a sprig of rosemary, alternatively you can take the arista, cover it with slices of bacon and tie it with string.

Also insert a sprig of rosemary in the twine, then salt, pepper and massage the meat to season it. Wash and trim the zucchini. Now heat the olive oil with two peeled garlic cloves in a pan.

Lay the arista and let it brown on all sides for a couple of minutes so that it seals well, once it is golden on the surface, blend with the white wine and let the alcohol evaporate. At this point transfer the arista to a baking tray.

Pour the baby zucchini into the pan with the meat's cooking liquid, cover with 30 g of water, salt and sauté the zucchini for 1 minute. Turn off the heat, remove the garlic 8 and transfer the zucchini and the cooking liquid into the pan with the arista. Cook in a static preheated oven at 170° for about 60-70 minutes: insert a probe into the meat to measure the internal temperature, which must reach 68° for optimal cooking.

While the meat is cooking, take care of the cherry tomato compote: wash and cut the cherry tomatoes in half, clean and slice the red onion, pour the cherry tomatoes into a small pot together with the onion.

Add the sugar, white wine vinegar and cook over medium-high heat for about 30 minutes, halfway through cooking season with chilli pepper and salt.

At the end of cooking the tomatoes will be soft and not too dry. Once the meat is cooked, remove the string with scissors, slice the meat and serve it with the zucchini and cherry tomato compote, season the dish with thyme.

STORAGE

You can keep the arista with cherry tomato jam in the refrigerator for 2 days, in a hermetically sealed container. You can freeze it if you have used fresh ingredients not thawed once cooked and completely cooled, maybe sliced to thaw only the part you need.

BAKED SALMON IN GINGER CRUST

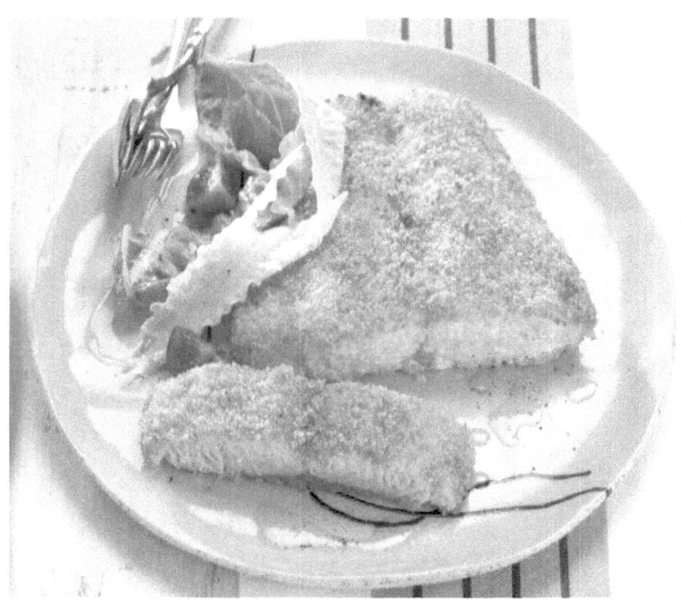

Ingredients

- 800 gr salmon fillet

- 100 gr breadcrumbs

- 5 cm ginger

- 2 spring onion

- extra virgin olive oil

- salt

Prepare the ginger. Peel and slice a small piece of ginger root about 2 inches long. Put it in the blender jar with 100 g of breadcrumbs and a generous pinch of salt.

Clean the spring onions. Cut off the root and the green end of the 2 spring onions, wash them and slice them thinly.

Put the spring onions in a blender with the other ingredients, add 6-7 tablespoons of oil and blend until a smooth cream is obtained.

Spread the salmon. Remove any bones from the salmon fillet with the help of tweezers, wash and dry it. Place it on the baking sheet lined with baking paper and cover it evenly with the prepared cream. Turn on the grill and, when it is hot, put the plate halfway up in the oven.

Bake the salmon in the oven for about 10 minutes, until a crunchy golden crust has formed on the surface.

CONCLUSIONI

Thank you for making it through to the end of this book, let's hope it was informative and able to provide you with all the tools you need to achieve your goals whatever they may be.

This book has tried to bring all the important points to the fore so that you can get all the information you need and the benefits of natural products without having to deal with their negative effects.

It is always advisable to consult a doctor in case of prolonged post-operative recovery phases.

I hope that this book can help you in achieving your goals.

Finally, if you found this book useful in any way, a review on Amazon is always appreciated!

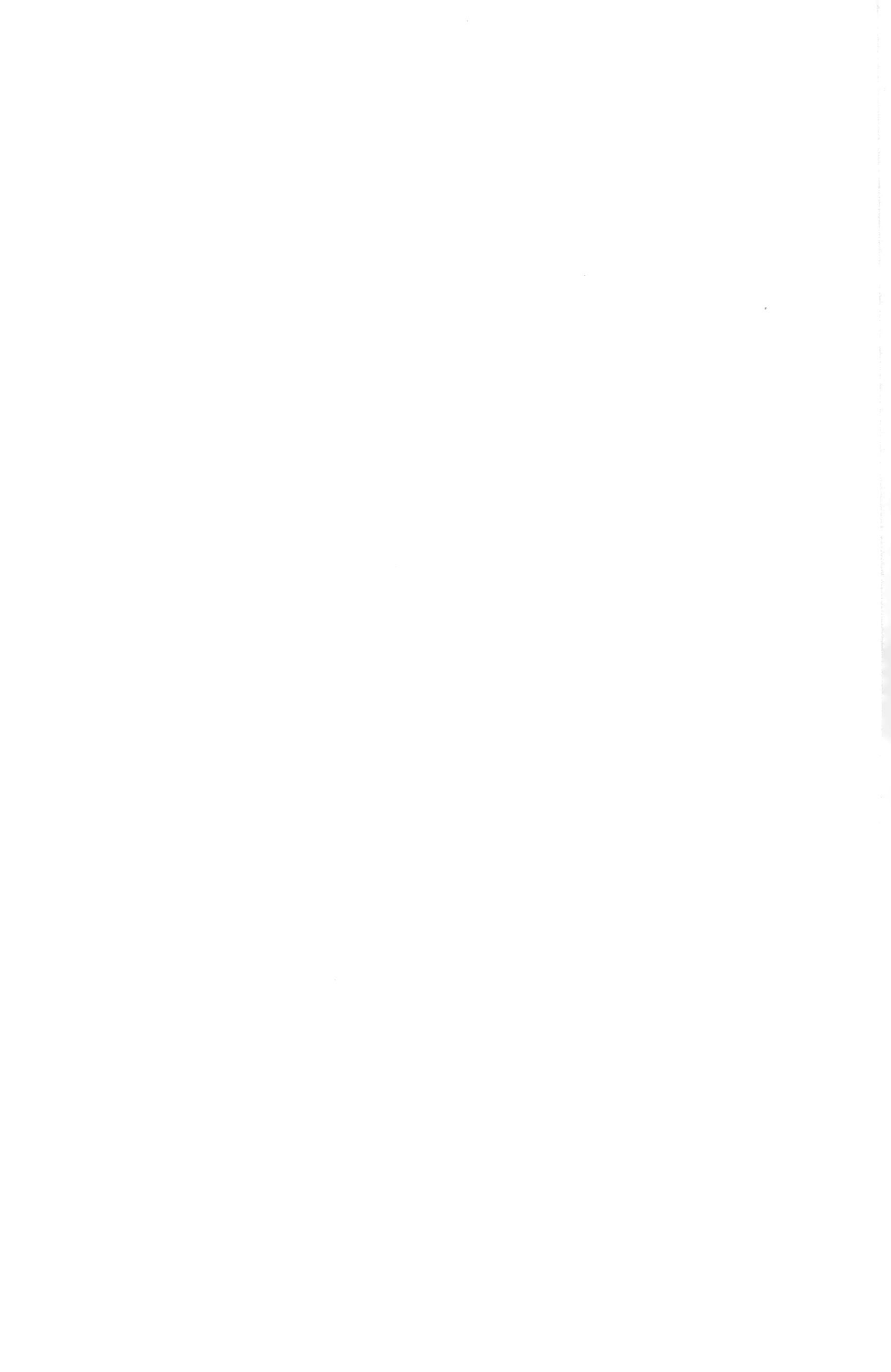